Take
Control

Navigating the challenges of living with an Aortic Aneurysm for People over 60.

SCOTT SCHMIDT

Learning to live with heart disease.

Forward

Embracing Change - A Journey Through Aortic Aneurysm

Life has a way of catapulting us into uncharted territories, often leaving us no choice but to navigate the unknown with courage and resilience. For me, that pivotal moment arrived on the day I received a diagnosis that changed the trajectory of my life: an aortic aneurysm.

As I sat in the cardiologist's office, absorbing the weight of those words, the world seemed to stand still. The doctor's explanation of the condition was accompanied by a palpable absence of guidance or resources, leaving me to grapple with the uncertainty of this medical journey alone. It was a daunting prospect, but little did I know that this moment would become the catalyst for a profound transformation.

Faced with the challenge of understanding and managing an aortic aneurysm, I turned to the one tool that has revolutionized the way we access information: the internet. In the vast sea of online resources, I began my journey of self-education. What started as a quest for basic knowledge evolved into a deep dive into the intricacies of aortic health, from understanding the mechanics of an aneurysm to exploring ways to prevent its growth.

This book is not just a compilation of facts and figures; it's a chronicle of my personal odyssey. A journey marked by the highs of empowerment and the lows of frustration, as I sought to reclaim control over my health and well-being. With every click, every article read, and every expert consulted, I discovered the profound impact that lifestyle choices can have on managing and mitigating the effects of an aortic aneurysm.

In these pages, I share not only the knowledge I've gained but the emotional and physical struggles I've faced. From dietary changes to tailored exercise regimens, I found a path that allowed me to live a fulfilling life while keeping my condition in check. This book is a testament to the resilience of the human spirit and the transformative power of knowledge.

My hope is that by sharing my story, I can provide a beacon of hope for those who find themselves navigating the uncertain waters of aortic health. May this book be a guide, a companion, and a source of inspiration for anyone facing the challenges of an aortic aneurysm. Together, let us embrace change, armed with information, courage, and the belief that life, even in the face of adversity, is a journey worth living to the fullest.

CONTENTS

Chapter One

Introduction

Embracing Wellness: A Gentle Journey to Health After 60

Welcome to a transformative journey towards wellness and vitality tailored specifically for individuals over 60 who navigate the challenges of living with an Aortic Aneurysm. This book is more than a guide; it's an invitation to reclaim control over your health and embrace a lifestyle centered around gentle, low-impact exercises.

A Personal Journey

As the author of this guide, I understand the unique concerns and aspirations that accompany aging, especially when faced with health conditions like Aortic Aneurysm. My own journey, coupled with the experiences of countless individuals I've encountered, has inspired the creation of this resource.

The Power of Movement

In the pages that follow, we embark on a journey together—one that celebrates the incredible potential of our bodies and the healing power of mindful movement. Whether you're seeking to manage Aortic Aneurysm, enhance your cardiovascular health, or simply stay active and vibrant, this book is crafted with your well-being in mind.

Navigating Exercise After 60

Exercise is a cornerstone of a healthy lifestyle, yet the approach must be thoughtful, especially as we age. This guide is designed for those who understand the importance of staying active but are mindful of the unique considerations that come with the presence of an Aortic Aneurysm.

What to Expect

In the upcoming chapters, we'll explore the fundamentals of Aortic Aneurysm, providing you with insights that empower informed decision-making. We'll then dive into a carefully crafted low-impact exercise program, emphasizing cardiovascular health, joint protection, and overall well-being.

A Journey of Empowerment

Consider this book your companion, offering guidance, encouragement, and a roadmap to a healthier, more vibrant life. Each chapter is a step forward on your journey of self-discovery and empowerment.

Track Your Progress

I have always enjoyed data and tracking results over time. It was easy for me to set up a simple chart to track my own success. Below is one of the charts I used on my journey. Email me if you would like a copy of this chart.

	30 Days	60 Days	90 Days	120 Days	150 Days	180 Days	210 Days	240 Days	270 Days	300 Days	330 Days	360 Days
Date:												
Weight:												
Resting Heart Rate:												
Blood Pressure - Systolic:												
Blood Pressure - Dystolic:												
Waist Size:												

Before We Begin

Before we embark on this transformative journey, remember that safety is paramount. Always consult with your healthcare provider before initiating any new exercise program. This guide is not a substitute for professional medical advice but rather a tool to complement your overall well-being strategy.

Are you ready to embrace wellness, celebrate movement, and embark on a journey to a healthier you? Let's take the first step together.

NOTES:

Chapter Two

Aortic Aneurysm Basics

What is an Aortic Aneurysm?

Understanding your body and the conditions it may face is a crucial step toward maintaining optimal health. In this chapter, we will delve into the basics of Aortic Aneurysm, shedding light on what happens within our bodies and why it's essential to approach exercise with care when managing this condition.

The Marvel of the Aorta

At the heart of our circulatory system lies the aorta, a remarkable vessel responsible for carrying oxygenated blood from the heart to the rest of the body. Think of it as the body's grand central highway, ensuring that every organ and tissue receives the vital nourishment it needs.

Aortic Aneurysm Unveiled

Now, imagine a weakened section along this grand highway, a ballooning or swelling known as an Aortic Aneurysm. This abnormal bulge can occur in either the abdominal or thoracic region of the aorta, presenting unique challenges and considerations.

The Types of Aortic Aneurysms

Abdominal Aortic Aneurysm (AAA):

This type affects the lower part of the aorta, typically occurring below the kidneys. Understanding AAA is crucial as it may influence the types of exercises that are suitable for your condition.

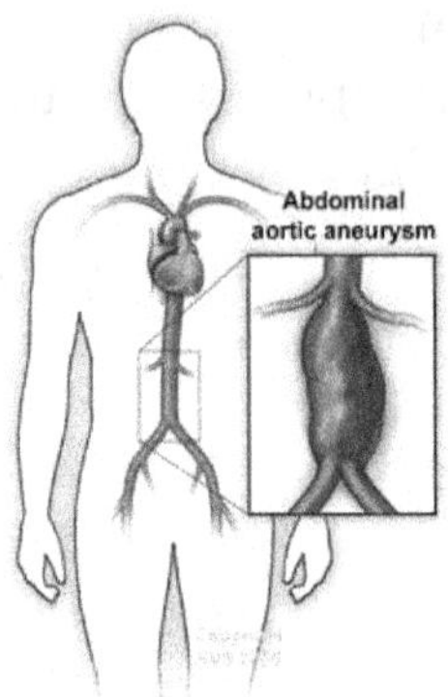

Image from Society for Vascular Surgery

Thoracic Aortic Aneurysm (TAA):

In contrast, TAA involves the upper part of the aorta that runs through the chest. The location of the aneurysm can impact the symptoms experienced and the approach to exercise.

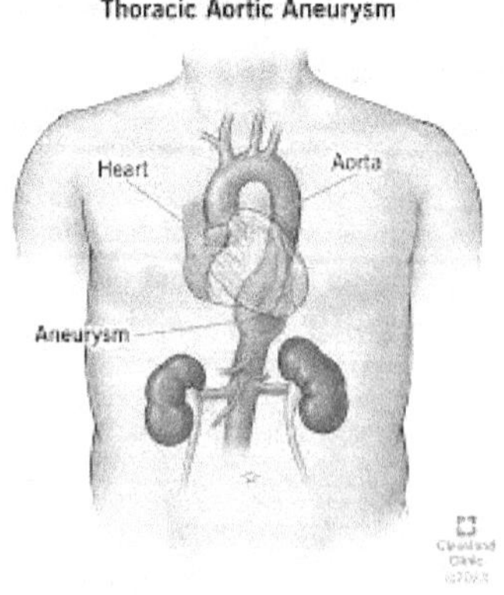

Image from Cleveland Clinic

The Heart of the Matter

During an Aortic Aneurysm, the weakened wall of the aorta may progressively expand, potentially leading to a rupture—a severe and life-threatening event. However, not all aneurysms progress to this point, and many can be managed with a combination of medical care, lifestyle adjustments, and, importantly, exercise.

Exercise Considerations

As we explore the benefits of low-impact exercises in later chapters, it's essential to grasp the fundamentals of the Aortic Aneurysm. This knowledge will empower you to make informed decisions about the types and intensity of exercises that align with your specific situation.

In the following sections, we'll discuss the distinctive features of abdominal and thoracic aortic aneurysms, providing you with a foundation to tailor your exercise routine to your unique needs. Remember, knowledge is a powerful tool, and by understanding the basics of Aortic Aneurysm, you take the first step towards a healthier and more informed lifestyle.

Chapter Three

Benefits of Low-Impact Exercise

Cardiovascular Health: Nourishing Your Heart with Gentle Motion

Our hearts are resilient, beating tirelessly to sustain life. In this chapter, we explore the profound impact of low-impact exercises on cardiovascular health, outlining how these gentle movements can become the foundation for a stronger and more resilient heart.

The Heart's Dance

Picture your heart as a rhythmic dancer, orchestrating the symphony of blood circulation. Cardiovascular health is paramount, especially when managing conditions like Aortic Aneurysm. Engaging in low-impact exercises sets the stage for a harmonious dance, promoting blood flow, and enhancing the efficiency of your circulatory system.

Low-Impact Aerobics: A Heart-Healthy Symphony

Aerobic exercises are the heartbeat of any fitness routine. In this section, we'll explore low-impact options such as brisk walking, swimming, and stationary cycling. These activities elevate your heart rate without subjecting your body to excessive strain, fostering cardiovascular endurance and resilience.

Joint Protection: Preserving Your Body's Foundation

As we age, our joints, the pillars supporting our bodies, require careful attention. Low-impact exercises become gentle architects, preserving joint health and mobility. In this chapter, we'll uncover how these exercises provide the perfect balance—nourishing your heart while safeguarding your joints.

The Art of Low-Impact Strength Training

Strength training, often associated with lifting heavy weights, takes on a new, gentle form in our low-impact exercise journey. We'll explore bodyweight exercises and resistance techniques that not only build strength but do so with a mindful approach, ensuring the safety of your joints and the overall well-being of your body.

Overall Well-being: Nurturing Body and Mind

Physical health is intricately linked to mental and emotional well-being. Low-impact exercises go beyond the physical realm, offering a holistic approach to health. Join us as we delve into the profound impact of these exercises on your mood, cognitive function, and overall quality of life.

The Mind-Body Connection

Discover the intimate connection between physical activity and mental health. Learn how low-impact exercises release endorphins, the body's natural mood elevators, and contribute to a positive mindset. As we navigate the terrain of overall well-being, you'll uncover the transformative power of exercise on your entire being.

In the chapters that follow, we'll embark on a practical journey, outlining specific low-impact exercises tailored to promote cardiovascular health, protect your joints, and enhance your overall well-being. Remember, each movement is a step towards a healthier, more vibrant you.

Chapter Four

Exercise Program Overview

Introduction:

In Chapter 4, we delve into the crucial aspect of your exercise program—the warm-up. A proper warm-up sets the tone for a safe and effective workout by preparing your body for the physical demands ahead. Following the warm-up, we explore a variety of low-impact aerobic exercises to enhance cardiovascular health and endurance. Additionally, we introduce gentle strength training exercises that focus on body weight or light resistance to maintain and improve overall muscle strength.

Before commencing this or any exercise program, it is advisable to consider acquiring an exercise watch or heart rate monitor that can be regularly consulted during your workout sessions. Prior to initiating any fitness regimen, it is strongly recommended to consult with your doctor or cardiologist for guidance and advice regarding appropriate heart rate ranges for low-impact exercises.

Warm-up: Preparing Your Body for Motion

The Importance of a Proper Warm-up

Before embarking on any exercise journey, it's crucial to lay the foundation with a thoughtful warm-up. This phase isn't just a preamble; it's a vital component in injury prevention and optimizing your body for the challenges ahead. A proper warm-up increases blood flow, warms up muscles, and enhances flexibility, setting the stage for a safe and effective workout.

Low-Impact Warm-up Exercises

Let's initiate our exercise routine with a series of low-impact warm-up exercises, designed with the unique needs of individuals with Aortic Aneurysm in mind. These movements focus on gentle joint mobilization, gradually elevating your heart rate, and preparing your body for the rhythmic journey ahead.

Before engaging in any physical activity, it is essential to dedicate time to warming up your body. This not only helps prevent injury but also optimizes your performance during the main exercise routine. Below are some low-impact warm-up exercises designed to get your blood flowing and muscles ready for action:

Joint Mobilization Exercises:

- Neck rotations
- Shoulder circles
- Hip circles
- Ankle rolls

Cardiovascular Warm-up:

- Light jogging in place
- Jumping jacks
- High knees
- Arm swings

Dynamic Stretching:

- Leg swings
- Arm circles
- Torso twists
- Walking lunges

Remember, the warm-up should last about 5-10 minutes, gradually increasing in intensity to elevate your heart rate and warm up major muscle groups.

Aerobic Exercises: Nourishing Your Heart with Motion

The Cardiovascular Benefits of Aerobic Exercise

Imagine your heart as a resilient maestro leading a symphony of health. Aerobic exercises are the heartbeat of this symphony, contributing to cardiovascular well-being. Engaging in regular, low-impact aerobic activities not only enhance heart health but also fortifies your stamina, providing the energy needed for the dance of life.

Low-Impact Aerobic Options

Our journey into aerobic exercise introduces you to a range of low-impact options. From the simplicity of walking to the fluidity of swimming and the accessibility of stationary cycling, we'll explore activities that elevate your heart rate without overburdening your body. Every step is a beat, orchestrating a harmonious balance between exertion and comfort.

Aerobic exercises play a pivotal role in enhancing cardiovascular health and promoting overall well-being. The following low-impact aerobic exercises provide options suitable for various fitness levels:

Walking: Brisk walking in your neighborhood or on a treadmill.

Swimming: Gentle laps or water aerobics for a full-body workout with minimal impact.

| **Stationary Cycling:** | Riding a stationary bike to improve cardiovascular endurance without stressing joints. |

| **Elliptical Trainer:** | Mimicking the motion of running without impacting your joints. |

| **Dance Aerobics:** | Enjoyable and rhythmic movements to boost heart rate and coordination. |

Each of these exercises can be adapted to your fitness level, making them accessible and enjoyable for everyone.

Strength Training:

Maintaining muscle strength is fundamental for overall health and functionality. The following gentle strength training exercises can be incorporated into your routine using either body weight or light resistance:

Bodyweight Squats: Strengthening your lower body muscles.

Push-ups: Building upper body strength and stability. You can also do standing push-ups against a wall.

Plank: Engaging core muscles for stability and strength.

Dumbbell Exercises: Incorporating light dumbbells for bicep curls, lateral raises, and tricep extensions.

Resistance Band Work: Utilizing resistance bands for added challenge in exercises like leg press and rows.

These strength exercises, performed 2-3 times a week, contribute to maintaining and enhancing muscle mass, which is crucial for supporting daily activities and preventing age-related muscle loss.

In summary, a well-rounded warm-up, coupled with a variety of low-impact aerobic exercises and gentle strength training, forms the foundation of your exercise program. This holistic approach ensures a balanced and sustainable fitness routine that contributes to your overall health and well-being.

NOTES:

Chapter Five

Flexibility and Balance

Flexibility Exercises: Preserving Joint Mobility

The Significance of Flexibility in Aging

As the clock ticks, maintaining the flexibility of your joints becomes paramount. Joint mobility is the key to graceful aging, and our flexibility exercises are tailored to preserve this essential element of your well-being. These gentle stretches not only foster flexibility but also encourage a sense of liberation in your movements.

Low-Impact Flexibility Routines

Join us in the exploration of low-impact flexibility routines. Each stretch is an invitation to honor your body, encouraging suppleness and range of motion. With deliberate, controlled movements, you'll embark on a journey to unlock the full potential of your body while safeguarding against undue strain.

Flexibility Exercises:

1. **Neck Stretch:**

   This exercise aims to alleviate tension in the neck and upper back, improving flexibility in cervical spine movement. Slow, controlled motions prevent strain.

2. **Shoulder Stretch:**

   Crossing one arm over the chest engages the shoulder muscles and promotes flexibility in the shoulder joint, vital for maintaining range of motion.

3. **Seated Forward Bend:**

Focusing on the hamstrings and lower back, this stretch enhances flexibility in the posterior chain, aiding in posture and reducing the risk of lower back discomfort.

4. **Hip Flexor Stretch:**

Targeting the hip flexors, this stretch improves flexibility in the hips, crucial for activities involving hip movement and preventing hip tightness.

5. **Calf Stretch:**

By stretching the calf muscles, this exercise supports ankle flexibility, important for activities like walking and running, and helps prevent calf tightness.

Role of Flexibility in Injury Prevention:

Flexibility plays a pivotal role in preventing injuries by allowing joints and muscles to move freely through their complete range of motion. Improved flexibility reduces the likelihood of strains, sprains, and other musculoskeletal injuries, especially important for individuals with Aortic Aneurysm to maintain overall physical health and well-being.

Balance Exercises:

1. **Single-Leg Stance:**

This exercise challenges and improves static balance, requiring engagement of core muscles and promoting stability. Progressing in duration enhances balance over time.

Purpose: The Single-Leg Stance is an exercise designed to challenge and improve static balance. It targets the core muscles, strengthens the stabilizing muscles around the hip and ankle joints, and enhances overall stability. Progressing in duration gradually over time helps to improve balance further.

Execution:

Starting Position: Stand on a flat surface with your feet hip-width apart. Engage your core muscles by pulling your belly button toward your spine. Shift your weight onto one leg.

Lift One Leg: Slowly lift the opposite foot off the ground, bringing the knee towards hip height. Keep the lifted foot flexed, with toes pointing forward. Find a focal point in front of you to help with balance.

Maintain Balance: Hold the single-leg position for as long as you can maintain good form. Focus on keeping your hips level and avoiding excessive tilting or swaying. Keep your standing knee slightly bent to avoid locking the joint.

Switch Legs: Lower the lifted foot back to the ground. Repeat the exercise on the opposite leg.

Tips: Begin with a short duration, aiming for 10-20 seconds on each leg. Gradually increase the time as your balance improves. Use a sturdy object, such as a chair or countertop, for support if needed. Focus on a spot at eye level to help stabilize your gaze and improve balance.

Progression: As you become more comfortable with the exercise, try closing your eyes to increase the challenge. Introduce small head turns or arm movements while maintaining balance. Incorporate variations, such as standing on a soft surface (e.g., a foam pad) to further engage stabilizing muscles.

Safety Considerations: Perform this exercise in a clear, open space to avoid obstacles. If using a support (chair or countertop), make sure it is stable and secure. If you have existing balance issues or medical concerns, consult with a healthcare professional before attempting this exercise.

The Single-Leg Stance is a simple yet effective exercise that can be incorporated into a daily routine to promote balance and stability. Regular practice can lead to improved proprioception and reduced risk of falls, especially important for individuals of all ages, including older adults.

2. **Heel-to-Toe Walk:**

Walking with a heel-to-toe motion enhances dynamic balance and coordination, mimicking real-world movements and improving gait stability.

Purpose: The Heel-to-Toe Walk is an exercise that focuses on enhancing dynamic balance and coordination. It mimics the natural heel-to-toe motion of walking, promoting gait stability and improving overall balance.

Execution:

Starting Position: Stand with your feet together, maintaining an upright posture. Place one foot in front of the other so that the heel of the front foot touches the toes of the back foot. Keep your gaze forward and engage your core muscles.

Walking Motion: Begin walking by lifting the back foot and placing it in front of the front foot. Ensure that the heel of the moving foot touches the toes of the stationary foot with each step. Maintain a smooth and controlled heel-to-toe motion.

Continue Forward: Continue walking in a straight line for a predetermined distance (e.g., 10-15 steps). Focus on a steady and deliberate pace, emphasizing the heel-to-toe movement.

Turn Around: When you reach the end of your chosen distance, pause, and turn around. Repeat the Heel-to-Toe Walk in the opposite direction.

Tips: Keep your eyes focused on a point in front of you to help maintain balance. Engage your core muscles to stabilize your body. Maintain a relaxed but controlled arm swing, similar to a natural walking motion. Pay attention to the placement of each foot, ensuring the heel touches the toe with each step.

Progression: Increase the challenge by walking on a narrow or uneven surface, such as a balance beam or grass. Introduce a head turn while walking to further challenge coordination. Gradually increase the walking distance as your balance improves.

Safety Considerations: Perform this exercise in a clear, open space to avoid obstacles. If needed, have a support such as a wall or countertop nearby for added stability. If you have existing balance issues or medical concerns, consult with a healthcare professional before attempting this exercise.

The Heel-to-Toe Walk is a practical exercise that incorporates real-world movements, making it beneficial for improving gait stability and coordination. It's suitable for individuals of various fitness levels and can be included as part of a balance and stability training routine.

3. **Balance Ball Exercises:**

Utilizing a stability ball adds an element of instability, requiring constant adjustments to maintain balance. These exercises engage core muscles and improve overall stability.

Purpose: Utilizing a stability ball adds an element of instability, requiring constant adjustments to maintain balance. These exercises engage core muscles and improve overall stability.

1. Ball Squats:

Purpose: Engages lower body muscles while challenging core stability.

Starting Position: Stand with your feet hip-width apart and place a stability ball between your lower back and a wall. Ensure the ball is at the small of your back, and your feet are positioned slightly in front.

Squatting Motion: Lower your body into a squat by bending your knees, keeping them in line with your toes. The ball rolls up the wall as you descend. Keep your back against the ball for support.

Return to Starting Position: Push through your heels and return to the starting position. Maintain engagement of your core throughout the exercise.

2. Plank with Ball Rollout:

Purpose: Targets the core, shoulders, and arms while challenging stability.

Starting Position: Begin in a plank position with your forearms on the stability ball and your toes on the ground. Maintain a straight line from head to heels.

Roll the Ball Out: Roll the stability ball away from your body by extending your arms. Keep your core tight to prevent your lower back from sagging.

Return to Plank: Use your core muscles to pull the ball back towards you, returning to the plank position. Ensure controlled movements to maximize stability benefits.

3. Ball Balance Exercise (Seated):

Purpose: Challenges core stability while seated.

Starting Position: Sit on the stability ball with your feet flat on the ground. Walk your feet forward, allowing the ball to roll until your back is comfortably supported.

Lift One Leg: Lift one foot off the ground, extending it forward. Maintain balance on the ball using your core muscles.

Alternate Legs: Lower the lifted foot and lift the other one. Continue alternating legs while keeping a stable seated position.

4. Lateral Ball Rolls:

Purpose: Targets the obliques and improves lateral stability.

Starting Position: Kneel on the ground with the stability ball to your side. Place your forearm on top of the ball, elbow directly beneath the shoulder.

Roll the Ball: Use your forearm to roll the ball away from your body while extending your legs into a side plank position. Keep your body in a straight line.

Return to Starting Position: Use your core muscles to pull the ball back towards you, returning to the starting position. Repeat on the other side.

Tips: Perform these exercises in a controlled manner to maximize the benefits of stability training. Focus on your breath and engage your core muscles throughout each exercise. Choose a stability ball size that allows you to maintain proper form.

Safety Considerations: Ensure the stability ball is properly inflated and in good condition. Perform exercises in a clear, open space to avoid collisions with objects. If you have existing stability issues or medical concerns, consult with a healthcare professional before attempting these exercises.

Incorporating these balance ball exercises into your routine can enhance core strength, stability, and overall balance. Gradually progress in difficulty as your stability improves, and always prioritize proper form and safety.

4. **Tai Chi Movements:**

Tai Chi emphasizes slow, deliberate movements, promoting mindfulness and enhancing balance, making it an excellent addition to the exercise program, particularly for individuals with Aortic Aneurysm. Here are a couple of easy Tai Chi Movements to get you started.

1. Ward Off (Peng):

Starting Position: Begin with your feet shoulder-width apart, knees slightly bent. Relax your shoulders and keep your arms in front of you, palms facing down.

Movement: Shift your weight to one leg as you gently raise your arms, palms turning upward. Imagine pushing away any tension or negative energy as your hands move forward. Shift your weight back to the center and repeat on the other side.

2. Grasp the Sparrow's Tail (Lan Que Wei):

Starting Position: Stand with feet shoulder-width apart, knees slightly bent.

Raise your arms to chest level, palms facing each other.

Movement: Begin by turning to one side, allowing your arms to follow the movement. As you turn, let one hand extend forward and the other hand move to the side. Imagine gently grasping and guiding the sparrow with your extended hand. Repeat on the other side.

3. Wave Hands Like Clouds (Yun Shou):

Starting Position: Stand with feet shoulder-width apart, knees slightly bent. Hold your arms in front of you, palms facing each other, as if holding a ball.

Movement: Shift your weight to one side and allow your arms to follow the movement. Imagine your hands floating through the air like clouds. Smoothly transition to the other side, creating a continuous, flowing motion.

4. Brush Knee and Twist Step (Lou Xi Ao Bu):

Starting Position: Stand with feet shoulder-width apart. Extend one foot forward and slightly to the side.

Movement: Shift your weight onto the forward foot. As you do, raise one arm, and imagine brushing your knee with the opposite hand. Twist your torso gently to face the forward foot.

5. Single Whip (Dan Bian):

Starting Position: Begin with your feet shoulder-width apart and knees slightly bent. Hold your arms in front of you, palms facing down.

Movement: Shift your weight to one side and extend the opposite arm to the side. The extended arm forms a soft and flowing arc, creating a "whip" motion. The other hand remains in front of you, palm facing down.

6. Closing Form (He Qi):

Starting Position: Stand with feet shoulder-width apart, knees slightly bent.

Bring your palms together in front of your chest, fingers pointing upward.

Movement: Slowly lower your hands, symbolizing the conclusion of the Tai Chi routine. Focus on your breath, inhaling and exhaling deeply. Maintain a relaxed and centered posture.

Tips: Move slowly and with intention, paying attention to your body and breath. Keep your movements smooth and continuous. Adapt the movements based on your comfort level and avoid overexertion.

These Tai Chi movements are just a small sample, and there are many more forms and variations to explore. Consistent practice can bring about numerous physical and mental benefits, promoting relaxation and balance. Always listen to your body, progress at your own pace, and consult with a healthcare professional if you have specific health concerns or conditions.

Importance of Balance Exercises:

Enhanced balance is crucial for preventing falls, especially significant for individuals with Aortic Aneurysm, as it reduces the risk of accidents and supports overall coordination. These exercises contribute to functional fitness, aiding in daily activities and reducing the likelihood of injuries related to loss of balance.

Chapter Six

Cool-Down and Recovery

Cool-Down Routine: Easing Your Body Gradually

The Purpose of a Cool-Down

As the curtains draw to a close on your exercise routine, the cool-down takes center stage. This phase is not merely a conclusion; it's a deliberate transition that eases your body from heightened activity to a state of calm. A proper cool-down is your post-workout ritual, reducing muscle tension, preventing soreness, and signaling the body that it's time to unwind.

Low-Impact Cool-Down Exercises

Join us in the serene world of low-impact cool-down exercises. These movements are designed to be soothing and meditative, promoting relaxation and restoring your body's equilibrium. As you gracefully guide your body through each motion, you embark on a journey of restoration, allowing your heart rate to gently descend and your muscles to surrender to tranquility.

Cool-Down Routine:

1. **Slow Walking or Marching in Place:**

    Gradually reducing the intensity of movement allows the heart rate to decrease gradually, preventing sudden drops in blood pressure and minimizing the risk of dizziness.

2. **Gentle Stretching:**

    Performing static stretches during the cool-down helps maintain and improve flexibility, reducing muscle stiffness and soreness post-exercise.

3. **Deep Breathing Exercises:**

   Deep breathing promotes relaxation and helps shift the body from a state of heightened activity to a more restful state, aiding in overall recovery.

Importance of Cool-Down:

A proper cool-down routine is essential for transitioning the body from a state of exertion to rest. It assists in preventing muscle soreness, reduces the risk of injury, and promotes flexibility, contributing to the overall effectiveness of the exercise program.

Recovery Tips:

Hydration:

Rehydration is crucial to replace fluids lost through sweat during exercise, supporting optimal physiological function and recovery.

Nutrition:

Consuming a balanced meal or snack with a combination of protein and carbohydrates aids in muscle recovery, replenishing energy stores, and supporting overall health.

Rest:

Adequate sleep is essential for recovery, as it allows the body to repair and regenerate tissues, contributing to improved performance and overall well-being.

Role of Recovery in Exercise Program:

Post-exercise recovery is a key component of the exercise program. Proper recovery strategies optimize performance, reduce the risk of overtraining, and contribute to long-term fitness gains and overall well-being.

Chapter Seven

Exercise Descriptions And Modifications

Exercise Descriptions: Guiding Your Movement

Detailed Instructions for Each Exercise

Welcome to the heart of your exercise program, where each movement is a carefully choreographed step towards your well-being. In this section, you'll find detailed instructions for every exercise. Clear, concise guidance will empower you to navigate each motion with confidence, ensuring proper form and maximizing the benefits of your efforts.

Modifications: Tailoring the Program to Your Needs

Variations for Different Fitness Levels

In the tapestry of fitness, one size does not fit all. This chapter introduces modifications tailored to different fitness levels. Whether you're taking your first steps into exercise or you're an experienced enthusiast, these variations ensure that the program is accessible and adaptable, accommodating everyone on their unique fitness journey.

Individuals with Aortic Aneurysm:

Specific modifications are provided to address the unique considerations of individuals with Aortic Aneurysm, ensuring a safe and tailored exercise program.

Different Fitness Levels:

Variations for different fitness levels are included to accommodate beginners, intermediate, and advanced participants, promoting inclusivity and scalability.

Exercise Descriptions:

Accompanying the program are detailed instructions and visuals for each exercise. These provide clarity on proper form, execution, and the targeted muscle groups, ensuring participants perform each exercise correctly.

Low-Impact Warm-up Exercises

1. Neck Rotations:

Purpose: Neck rotations help improve the flexibility of the cervical spine and reduce stiffness in the neck muscles.

Execution: Sit or stand with a straight spine and relaxed shoulders. Slowly turn your head to one side, bringing your chin towards your shoulder. Hold the position for 5-10 seconds, feeling a gentle stretch in the neck. Return your head to the center. Repeat the movement on the opposite side.

Perform 8-10 repetitions on each side.

Tips: Move your head in a smooth, controlled manner. Avoid jerky or forceful movements. Do not rotate your head beyond a comfortable range.

2. Shoulder Circles:

Purpose: Shoulder circles help improve mobility in the shoulder joints and reduce tension in the surrounding muscles.

Execution: Stand with your feet shoulder-width apart. Lift your shoulders towards your ears in a shrugging motion. Rotate your shoulders backward in a circular motion.

Complete 8-10 rotations in one direction.

Reverse the direction and perform 8-10 rotations in the opposite direction.

Tips: Keep your movements slow and controlled. Engage your core muscles to maintain stability. Relax your neck and jaw during the exercise.

3. Hip Circles:

Purpose: Hip circles enhance flexibility in the hip joints and help improve overall hip mobility.

Execution: Stand with your feet hip-width apart. Place your hands on your hips. Rotate your hips in a circular motion, moving them forward, to the side, backward, and then to the other side.

Complete 8-10 rotations in one direction.

Reverse the direction and perform 8-10 rotations in the opposite direction.

Tips: Keep your knees slightly bent throughout the exercise. Engage your core muscles to support your lower back. Perform the movements smoothly without any sudden jerks.

4. Ankle Rolls:

Purpose: Ankle rolls help improve ankle joint mobility and flexibility, and they can be beneficial for those with ankle stiffness.

Execution: Sit or stand with your feet flat on the ground. Lift one foot slightly off the ground. Rotate your ankle in a circular motion, moving it clockwise for 8-10 rotations. Reverse the direction and rotate the ankle counterclockwise for 8-10 rotations. Switch to the other ankle and repeat the process.

Tips: Perform the rotations in a controlled manner. Keep your movements within a pain-free range. Do not force the ankles into uncomfortable positions.

Cardiovascular Warm-up:

1. Light Jogging in Place:

Purpose: Light jogging in place serves as a warm-up activity to increase heart rate, warm up muscles, and prepare the cardiovascular system for more intense physical activity.

Execution: Stand with your feet hip-width apart. Begin jogging in place, lifting your knees towards your chest and keeping a light, bouncy motion. Swing your arms naturally in coordination with your leg movements. Maintain a brisk but comfortable pace. Continue for 2-5 minutes as part of your warm-up routine.

Tips: Land softly on the balls of your feet to minimize impact. Gradually increase the intensity as your body warms up. Keep your upper body relaxed and maintain good posture.

2. Jumping Jacks:

Purpose: Jumping jacks are a full-body exercise that helps improve cardiovascular fitness, coordination, and overall muscle engagement.

Execution: Start in a standing position with your feet together and arms at your sides. Jump your feet out to the sides while simultaneously raising your arms overhead. Jump back to the starting position, bringing your arms back down to your sides. Repeat the motion in a rhythmic and continuous manner. Aim for 1-2 minutes as part of a cardio workout or warm-up.

Tips: Land softly with slightly bent knees to reduce impact. Engage your core muscles to stabilize your body. Maintain a steady pace for the duration of the exercise.

3. High Knees:

Purpose: High knees are an effective exercise for increasing heart rate, warming up the lower body, and improving coordination and endurance.

Execution: Stand with your feet hip-width apart. Lift one knee towards your chest as high as comfortably possible. Quickly switch and lift the other knee, creating a running-in-place motion. Swing your arms in coordination with your leg movements. Continue at a brisk pace for 1-2 minutes.

Tips: Land on the balls of your feet with each knee lift. Maintain an upright posture and engage your core. Focus on lifting your knees as high as possible for maximum benefit.

4. Arm Swings:

Purpose: Arm swings help to improve shoulder mobility, warm up the upper body, and increase blood flow to the arms.

Execution: Stand with your feet shoulder-width apart. Extend your arms straight out to the sides. Swing your arms in small circles, gradually increasing the size of the circles. After 10-15 seconds, reverse the direction of the arm swings. Continue for 1-2 minutes, gradually incorporating different arm movements.

Tips: Keep your movements controlled to avoid strain. Focus on a full range of motion in the shoulder joints. Incorporate variations, such as forward and backward arm swings, to target different muscles.

Dynamic Stretching:

1. Leg Swings:

Purpose: Leg swings are dynamic stretches that target the hip flexors, hamstrings, and quadriceps, improving flexibility and increasing blood flow to the lower body.

Execution: Stand next to a support (such as a wall or a sturdy pole) for balance. Swing one leg forward and backward in a controlled manner. After completing the forward swings, swing the leg sideways, crossing the midline of the body. Repeat the same motions with the other leg. Perform 10-15 swings for each leg in each direction.

Tips: Keep your torso upright and engage your core for stability. Perform the swings with a gradual and controlled motion. Do not force the leg beyond a comfortable range of motion.

2. Arm Circles:

Purpose: Arm circles help to warm up the shoulder joints, improve flexibility, and increase blood flow to the arms.

Execution: Stand with your feet shoulder-width apart. Extend your arms straight out to the sides. Begin making circular motions with your arms, gradually increasing the size of the circles. After 10-15 seconds, reverse the direction of the arm circles. Continue for 1-2 minutes, focusing on a full range of motion.

Tips: Keep your movements controlled to avoid strain. Engage your core muscles for stability. Gradually increase the size of the circles as your shoulders warm up.

3. Torso Twists:

Purpose: Torso twists engage the muscles of the core, spine, and hips, promoting flexibility and mobility in the upper body.

Execution: Stand with your feet shoulder-width apart. Place your hands on your hips or extend your arms straight in front of you. Twist your torso to one side, bringing your shoulders in the direction of your hip. Return to the center and then twist to the opposite side. Repeat the motion in a controlled manner, alternating sides. Perform 10-15 twists on each side.

Tips: Keep your hips facing forward throughout the movement. Engage your abdominal muscles as you twist. Move slowly and avoid any sudden or jerky motions.

4. Walking Lunges:

Purpose: Walking lunges are effective for warming up the lower body, targeting the quadriceps, hamstrings, and glutes while also improving balance and stability.

Execution: Start with your feet together. Take a step forward with one foot, lowering your body into a lunge position. The back knee should come close to the ground, and the front knee should be directly above the ankle. Push off the front foot to bring the back foot forward and into the next lunge. Continue walking forward, alternating legs with each step. Perform 10-15 lunges on each leg.

Tips: Keep your back straight and chest lifted. Engage your core for stability. Ensure that the front knee does not go beyond the toes.

These exercises can be incorporated into a dynamic warm-up routine before engaging in more intense physical activity. As always, listen to your body, modify exercises as needed, and consult with a fitness professional or healthcare provider if you have any concerns or health conditions.

Strength Training:

Bodyweight Squats:

Purpose: Bodyweight squats are a fundamental lower-body exercise that targets the muscles of the thighs, hips, and buttocks. This compound movement helps improve lower body strength, flexibility, and functional movement patterns.

Execution:

Starting Position: Stand with your feet shoulder-width apart. Keep your chest up, shoulders back, and gaze forward. Engage your core muscles for stability.

Squat Descent: Initiate the squat by pushing your hips back and bending your knees. Lower your body as if sitting back into an imaginary chair. Keep your back straight and chest lifted. Ensure your knees are in line with your toes, not extending beyond them.

Full Squat: Lower yourself until your thighs are parallel to the ground or as far as comfortably possible. Maintain a neutral spine throughout the movement.

Squat Ascent: Press through your heels and engage your glutes to return to the starting position. Straighten your legs and stand tall, squeezing your buttocks at the top.

Repetition: Perform the exercise in a controlled manner, focusing on proper form. Start with a manageable number of repetitions, such as 10-15, and gradually increase as your strength improves.

Tips:

Form is Key: Ensure proper form throughout the movement to prevent strain and injury.

Knee Alignment: Keep your knees in line with your toes and avoid letting them collapse inward.

Depth: Aim for a comfortable depth, gradually working towards a full range of motion.

Breathing: Inhale as you lower into the squat, exhale as you push back up.

Variations: As you progress, you can try different variations, such as sumo squats, pulsing squats, or adding a jump for more intensity.

Common Mistakes to Avoid: Allowing the knees to collapse inward. Rounding the back or leaning too far forward. Not going through a full range of motion. Using improper breathing techniques. Sacrificing form for the sake of speed.

Push-ups:

Purpose: Push-ups are a versatile and effective bodyweight exercise that primarily targets the muscles of the chest, shoulders, triceps, and core. They are a fundamental upper body strength exercise and contribute to overall upper body development.

Execution:

Starting Position: Begin in a plank position with your hands placed slightly wider than shoulder-width apart. Keep your wrists directly under your shoulders. Your body should form a straight line from head to heels.

Descent (Lowering Phase): Lower your body towards the ground by bending your elbows. Keep your body in a straight line without letting your hips sag or lift. Lower your chest until it almost touches the ground.

Full Extension: Push through your palms, straightening your arms to return to the starting position. Fully extend your arms without locking your elbows at the top.

Repetition: Perform the exercise in a controlled manner, maintaining proper form. Start with a number of repetitions that challenge you but allow for good form (e.g., 8-12 repetitions).

Tips:

Body Alignment: Maintain a straight line from head to heels throughout the movement.

Hand Placement: Hands slightly wider than shoulder-width, fingers pointing forward or slightly turned outward.

Elbow Position: Keep your elbows at a 45-degree angle to your body, not flaring out excessively.

Core Engagement: Tighten your core to keep your body stable.

Breathing: Inhale as you lower your body, exhale as you push back up.

Common Mistakes to Avoid: Allowing the lower back to sag or the hips to lift. Positioning hands too high or too low. Allowing the elbows to flare out excessively. Not lowering the chest close enough to the ground. Holding your breath during the exercise.

Progressions and Variations:

Incline Push-ups: Elevate your hands on a surface (e.g., a bench or a wall) to decrease the difficulty.

Decline Push-ups: Elevate your feet on a surface to increase the difficulty.

Diamond Push-ups: Place your hands close together beneath your chest to target triceps and inner chest.

Wide Grip Push-ups: Widen your hand placement to target the outer chest.

Plank:

Purpose: The plank is a foundational core exercise that targets the muscles of the abdomen, lower back, shoulders, and stabilizing muscles. It helps improve core strength, stability, and endurance.

Execution:

Starting Position: Begin in a prone position on the floor, facing down. Place your forearms on the ground, elbows directly beneath your shoulders. Keep your wrists parallel to the body, forming a 90-degree angle with your elbows. Extend your legs straight behind you, with toes on the ground.

Body Alignment: Engage your core muscles and maintain a straight line from your head to your heels. Avoid letting your hips sag or lifting them too high.

Hold Position: Hold the plank position for as long as you can maintain proper form. Focus on keeping your abdominal muscles tight and your body in a straight line.

Repetition: Perform the plank for a predetermined amount of time, such as 20-60 seconds. Gradually increase the duration as your strength and endurance improve.

Tips:

Neutral Spine: Keep your head in a neutral position, looking down at the ground.

Engage Core Muscles: Tighten your abdominal muscles and draw your navel towards your spine.

Breathing: Breathe deeply and evenly throughout the exercise.

Common Mistakes to Avoid: Allowing the lower back to sag or the hips to lift. Holding your breath instead of breathing regularly.

Letting the elbows move too far forward or backward. Not engaging the core muscles.

Variations:

High Plank: Similar to the standard plank, but with arms fully extended, hands directly beneath the shoulders.

Side Plank: Rotate your body to the side, balancing on one forearm and the side of your foot, forming a straight line from head to heels.

Plank with Shoulder Taps: In the plank position, lift one hand off the ground and tap the opposite shoulder, alternating sides.

Plank with Leg Lifts: Lift one leg off the ground while maintaining the plank position, alternating legs.

Progressions: Increase the duration of the plank. Add variations or combine it with other exercises in a circuit.

Dumbbell Exercises:

Using light dumbbells for these exercises is an excellent way to target specific muscle groups in the arms. Here's how you can perform each exercise:

1. Bicep Curls:

Purpose: Bicep curls primarily target the biceps brachii, which is the muscle on the front of your upper arm.

Execution: Stand with a dumbbell in each hand, arms fully extended, and palms facing forward. Keep your elbows close to your torso. Inhale and, while keeping your upper arms stationary, exhale as you curl the weights toward your shoulders. Hold the contracted position for a brief pause as you squeeze your biceps. Inhale and slowly begin to lower the dumbbells back to the starting position.

Tips: Perform the movement in a controlled manner to maximize muscle engagement. Avoid swinging the weights or using momentum. Keep your back straight and core engaged.

2. Lateral Raises:

Purpose: Lateral raises target the deltoid muscles, helping to sculpt the shoulders.

Execution: Stand with a dumbbell in each hand, arms by your sides, and palms facing your body. Maintain a slight bend in your elbows. Exhale and lift the weights out to the sides until your arms are parallel to the ground. Hold the contracted position for a brief pause. Inhale and slowly lower the dumbbells back to the starting position.

Tips: Use a controlled motion, avoiding any sudden jerks. Keep a slight bend in your elbows throughout the exercise. Focus on engaging the muscles of the shoulders.

3. Tricep Extensions:

Purpose: Tricep extensions target the triceps brachii, which is the muscle on the back of your upper arm.

Execution: Stand or sit with a dumbbell in one hand, arm fully extended overhead. Keep your elbow close to your head with your upper arm in a fixed position. Inhale and, while keeping your upper arm stationary, exhale as you lower the dumbbell behind your head. Hold the contracted position for a brief pause, feeling a stretch in your triceps. Inhale and slowly extend your arm, returning the dumbbell to the starting position.

Tips: Ensure that your elbow stays pointed upward throughout the movement. Use a weight that allows you to control the motion and maintain good form. Keep your core engaged for stability.

Sample Dumbbell Routine:

Bicep Curls: 3 sets of 12 reps.

Lateral Raises: 3 sets of 12 reps.

Tricep Extensions: 3 sets of 12 reps.

Rest between sets: 60 seconds.

Note: Adjust the weight of the dumbbells based on your fitness level and gradually increase as you gain strength. This sample routine can be incorporated into your overall strength training program for the arms. Always prioritize proper form and consult with a fitness professional or healthcare provider if you have specific concerns or conditions.

NOTES:

Chapter Eight

Safety Guidelines

Warning Signs: Listening to Your Body

Recognizing Signs to Stop Exercising

Your body is an intricate communicator, and paying attention to its signals is paramount. In this chapter, we explore the warning signs that may indicate it's time to pause your exercise journey. From subtle cues to more overt messages, understanding and heeding these signs will empower you to exercise safely and with mindful awareness.

Precautions: Exercising with Mindful Awareness

Exercise Precautions for Aortic Aneurysm

Safety is the cornerstone of our exercise program. This section outlines specific precautions to consider, especially when managing Aortic Aneurysm. By exercising with mindful awareness and embracing these precautions, you'll not only protect yourself but also foster a harmonious relationship between your body and the movements that nurture its well-being.

Warning Signs:

1. **Severe Chest Pain:**
   Intense chest pain during exercise may indicate a potential cardiac issue, warranting immediate cessation of activity and medical attention.

2. **Shortness of Breath:**

Severe or persistent shortness of breath could signal respiratory or cardiovascular issues, requiring prompt attention.

3. **Dizziness or Lightheadedness:**
Feeling dizzy or lightheaded may indicate dehydration, low blood sugar, or other issues. Stopping activity and resting is crucial.

Precautions:

1. **Consultation with a Healthcare Professional:**
Before starting the exercise program, consulting with a healthcare professional is essential, especially for individuals with Aortic Aneurysm, to ensure safety and suitability.
2. **Gradual Progression:**
Gradual progression in intensity and duration helps the body adapt to increased demands, reducing the risk of overexertion and injury.
3. **Monitoring Vital Signs:**
Regular monitoring of blood pressure and heart rate, both during and after exercise, provides insights into cardiovascular health and exercise tolerance.

Addressing Potential Contraindications:

Identifying and addressing any medical conditions or medications that may contraindicate specific exercises is crucial. Emphasizing the importance of personalized fitness programs and individualized precautions ensures participant safety and well-being.

Chapter Nine

Nutritional Tips

Balanced Nutrition: Fueling Your Active Lifestyle

The Role of Balanced Nutrition

As you embark on your journey to wellness, it's essential to recognize the symbiotic relationship between exercise and nutrition. Think of your body as a finely tuned machine—exercise propels it forward, while balanced nutrition provides the fuel. This section delves into the crucial role of a balanced diet in supporting your active lifestyle. From replenishing energy stores to aiding muscle recovery, the foods you choose play a vital role in optimizing your overall well-being.

Healthy Eating Habits

Let's unravel the principles of healthy eating that will complement your exercise routine seamlessly. We'll explore the importance of a well-rounded diet, emphasizing the inclusion of a variety of nutrient-dense foods. From whole grains and lean proteins to an abundance of fruits and vegetables, adopting healthy eating habits becomes an integral part of sustaining the newfound vitality that exercise brings.

Incorporate a Variety of Nutrients:

Diversifying your diet is a cornerstone of promoting overall health and well-being. Here's a closer look at the importance of incorporating a variety of nutrients:

Embarking on an active lifestyle demands a thoughtful approach to nutrition—one that encompasses a holistic understanding of the essential components supporting your overall well-being.

In this journey, consider the significance of:

Essential Vitamins and Minerals:

Include a diverse array of food types in your diet to ensure a rich spectrum of essential vitamins and minerals. These nutrients are not mere players; they orchestrate pivotal roles in various bodily functions, ranging from fortifying immune health to facilitating efficient energy metabolism.

Micronutrients for Optimal Function:

Different food groups offer a diverse array of micronutrients. Fruits and vegetables, for instance, bestow upon you a treasure trove of antioxidants, vitamins, and minerals that contribute to cellular health and act as guardians against disease.

Diverse Protein Sources:

Aim for a well-rounded mix of protein sources that includes lean meats, legumes, and plant-based options. Proteins, the architects of muscle repair, guardians of immune function, and custodians of cellular maintenance, are indispensable allies in your journey toward an active and vibrant lifestyle.

Healthy Fats:

Incorporate sources of healthy fats, such as avocados, nuts, and olive oil. These fats serve as champions for brain health, collaborators in hormone production, and facilitators in the absorption of fat-soluble vitamins.

Whole Grains:

Opt for whole grains over their refined counterparts to ensure a gradual and sustained release of energy. Whole grains bring a trio of benefits to the table—fiber for digestive health, B-vitamins for vitality, and antioxidants as guardians of your sustained energy levels.

This nuanced approach to nutrition, embracing a diverse range of nutrient sources, sets the stage for a harmonious relationship between your dietary choices and your active lifestyle. As you nourish your body with these essential elements, you lay the foundation for sustained vitality, resilience, and an overall sense of well-being.

Portion Control:

Understanding the role of portion control is fundamental to maintaining a healthy calorie balance and supporting overall wellness:

Navigating the realm of nutrition isn't solely about the foods you choose; it's also about how you engage with your meals. Consider the following principles for cultivating a mindful and balanced approach to eating:

Mindful Eating:

Embrace the practice of mindful eating by attuning yourself to the signals of hunger and fullness. This conscious approach to consuming food not only prevents overeating but also fosters a healthier relationship with what you eat. By paying attention to the nuances of your body's cues, you establish a profound connection between your mind and your nourishment.

Balanced Plate Approach:

Craft your meals with a balanced plate in mind, featuring appropriate servings of proteins, carbohydrates, and vegetables. This method ensures that each meal provides a harmonious blend of essential nutrients. By adopting the balanced plate approach, you create a foundation for sustained energy, supporting your active lifestyle with a robust nutritional framework.

Smaller, Well-Controlled Portions:

Delight in smaller portions of energy-dense foods to manage calorie intake without compromising on satisfaction. This approach, rooted in portion control, serves as a strategic ally in weight management, preventing the pitfalls of excessive caloric consumption. Enjoying your favorite foods in moderation becomes a key tenet of maintaining a balanced and sustainable relationship with nutrition.

Hydration with Meals:

Integrate hydration into your meals by sipping water throughout. This simple yet impactful practice enhances feelings of fullness, aiding in digestion and supporting overall metabolic processes. Staying adequately hydrated becomes a subtle yet influential component of your mindful eating journey, ensuring that your body operates optimally.

As you incorporate these mindful and balanced eating principles into your daily life, you cultivate not just a diet but a sustainable and harmonious approach to nourishment. Each meal becomes an opportunity to connect with your body, to savor the flavors, and to nourish yourself in a way that aligns with your active and vibrant lifestyle.

Stay Hydrated with Water-Rich Foods:

Navigating the realm of hydration goes beyond mere water intake—it's a holistic approach to supporting your overall health and well-being. Here's a closer look at key principles for embracing effective hydration:

The Importance of Hydration:

Understand the profound significance of hydration for your body's functions. Beyond quenching your thirst, proper hydration plays a crucial role in temperature regulation, nutrient transportation, and joint lubrication. This foundational aspect of well-being emphasizes the vital role water plays in maintaining the delicate balance within your body.

Water-Rich Foods for Dual Benefits:

Expand your hydration strategy by incorporating foods with high water content, such as watermelon, cucumbers, and oranges. These water-rich foods not only contribute to your hydration goals but also pack a nutritional punch, providing essential nutrients that enhance their overall value. This dual benefit underscores the synergy between hydration and optimal nutrition.

Strategic Hydration Choices:

Make mindful choices in your hydration routine by opting for beverages that align with your overall health goals. Choose hydrating options like herbal teas and infused water over sugary beverages. These choices not only contribute to your hydration needs but also reflect a conscious effort to support your body's well-being. This strategic approach to hydration elevates the practice from a mere routine to a thoughtful and health-conscious habit.

Balancing Electrolytes:

Consider the role of electrolytes in maintaining a delicate equilibrium within your body. Foods rich in electrolytes, such as coconut water and certain fruits, become valuable allies in sustaining this balance of essential minerals. By incorporating these electrolyte-rich foods into your diet, you contribute to the optimal functioning of your cells and support your body's intricate regulatory mechanisms.

In adopting these principles, hydration transforms from a basic necessity to a nuanced practice that enhances your overall health. Each sip and every water-rich bite becomes intentional choices, aligning with your commitment to well-being and providing your body with the essential support it needs to thrive.

Emphasis on the Role of Nutrition:

Proper nutrition is the cornerstone that sustains your body through the challenges of exercise and daily life. Here's a detailed exploration of its critical role:

Navigating the intricate relationship between nutrition and energy demands is key to optimizing your performance and supporting overall health. Let's delve into the principles that underscore the importance of fueling your body for the demands of exercise:

Fueling Energy Demands:

A well-balanced diet serves as the bedrock for meeting the energy demands of exercise. Among the macronutrients, carbohydrates take center stage as the primary energy source for physical activity. This section unveils the role of a balanced diet in providing the necessary fuel to power your movements, ensuring that your body is equipped to meet the demands of your exercise regimen.

Vitamins and Minerals for Performance:

Essential vitamins and minerals emerge as silent catalysts for optimizing performance. They contribute to the intricate dance of enzymes, muscle contractions, and oxygen transport, enhancing the overall efficiency of your exercise endeavors. This chapter unfolds the vital role that these micronutrients play in elevating your physical performance to new heights.

Preventing Fatigue:

Proper nutrition becomes a strategic ally in the battle against fatigue during and after exercise. Nutrient-dense meals and snacks form the foundation, ensuring that your body is equipped with the resources needed for sustained effort and efficient recovery. This section provides insights into the nutritional strategies that serve as guardians against the onset of fatigue, fostering a sense of endurance and resilience.

Supporting Immune Function:

Beyond the immediate realm of exercise, a well-balanced diet emerges as a fortifier of the immune system. This chapter explores how nutrients like vitamin C, zinc, and antioxidants play pivotal roles in supporting immune function. By nourishing your body with these immune-boosting elements, you not only reduce the risk of illness but also cultivate a foundation for robust overall health.

Maintaining Overall Health:

The journey of nutrition extends beyond the confines of exercise, influencing your overall health in profound ways. This section underscores the critical role of nutrition in maintaining cardiovascular health, bone density, and the prevention of chronic diseases. A diet rich in fruits, vegetables, lean proteins, and healthy fats becomes the cornerstone of a holistic approach to well-being.

In embracing these principles, you embark on a journey where nutrition isn't merely a complement to exercise—it's a dynamic force that powers your body, supports your performance, and lays the groundwork for enduring health and vitality.

In conclusion, understanding and implementing balanced nutrition is not just a component of your exercise program; it is the foundation for a healthy and vibrant life. It is a proactive investment in your well-being, ensuring that your body is equipped to thrive through the various demands and challenges it may encounter.

NOTES:

Chapter Ten

Motivation

Inspiring Transformations

My brother is 4 years older than me, and he is in great shape. He is a cross-fitter and spends time each day at the gym working on his health, but also on his mental health. I have witnessed the transition of people suffering from self-doubt and negative self-talk change over time as they show up each day to workout. When they push themselves and achieve daily, weekly, and monthly goals; the days of self-doubt and negative self-talk are replaced with self-confidence. They change from needing help and encouragement to providing the same to those just starting their journey. Planet Fitness charges $10/month for membership, and I recommend joining a local club and spending time around people who are working to be healthier and feed off their energy, positivity, and encouragement.

Words to Propel You Forward

It is easier to quit and give up when you don't put yourself out there. When you tell everyone what you're are working on, and then show up each day, you will find that the people in your life are your greatest cheerleaders. Don't be afraid to share and ask for help. You will find that there are so many people in this world who want to help but are waiting to be asked. As you take your journey, there will be those who encourage you and at some point, along your path, you will find that you are encouraging others just starting their journey. One day you will stop and look back and you'll realize you lost the person who started this journey and found someone new. A positive and encouraging person, not only at the gym, but in every aspect of your life, giving back to others.

Personal Struggle:

Up until my diagnosis with my aortic aneurism I was walking 10 miles a day as part of my work life. But as I started to make lifestyle changes because of the diagnoses I found myself slowing down. The 30-pound weight restriction and instructions from my cardiologist to stop if I felt I was putting any stress on my heart, along with the medications I was required to take really took a toll on me. I was tired all the time and found myself putting on weight because I had slowed down. It took me some time, a lot of research, and asking questions to find out what this diagnosis meant for me. I did have to make some changes and learn about living with an aortic aneurism, and about my lifestyle. Giving up something didn't mean I was less of the person I was, it just meant that I was becoming a better version of myself. Weight gain and tiredness were just a side effect of the disease and medication, not a reason for giving up. It was a driving force in uncovering my new lifestyle.

Transformations:

This isn't like a makeover, where you get a haircut, and new outfit and boom, you're done. This is an ongoing transformation you will work on for the rest of your life. You don't stop once you reach a goal, you update the goals and the path to achieving those goals, and then you get started again. If the goal is healthier eating, regular workouts, and lowering your heart rate and blood pressure. Then, once you reach that goal, the new goal is to maintain those numbers and activities. Such as finding new and fun ways to exercise. And, like myself, helping others who are just starting their journey, or who are struggling to find, or stay on their path.

Achievements:

Achievement results from effort. Consistent effort. This could include weight loss, improved fitness levels, enhanced mental well-being, becoming a healthier cook, or achieving fitness-related goals.

Celebrating these victories serves as a powerful motivator to reaching your next set of goals.

- ## Perseverance:

"It's not about how many times you fall but how many times you get back up." Setbacks are part of the journey. If you go on a trip and you run into a detour, do you stop and go home, or do you adjust your route and press on. The same should be true with your new journey. You **_WILL_** run into detours, but just recalculate and press on!

- ## Resilience:

"Strength does not come from the body; it comes from the will!" I love those videos of people who push themselves at marathons. You see them struggling to make it to the finish line. Pushing themselves despite the pain and misery they are feeling. Often, other runners will walk back, offering encouragement and in some cases a hand or shoulder to help them make it across the finish line. One specific video shows a woman who struggled to cross the line say after the race that she "didn't work for over a year to get to that race only to quit!" This is your LIFE, there is no quitting!

Rewards of Consistency:

Since I was a child, I have always had an interest in flying and with the space program. One of my favorite quotes is from NASA's Flight Director Gene Kranz, during the Apollo 13 Moon landing mission, when he said that "Failure is not an option!" The same holds true with us. Failure is not an option!

Encouragement:

Daily Affirmations:

Daily affirmations provide a proactive approach to maintaining a positive mindset. Crafting affirmations that resonate with your fitness goals and overall well-being is key.

- **Empowering Statements:**

  I have a deck of 3x5 cards with positive statements handwritten on them. "Do unto others as you would have them do unto you." Or "The last impression leaves a lasting impression." Or "Do your best, and then do a little more." Or "Leave people and places in better shape that when you found them!"

  These are the type of positive and empowering statements that help set the tone for your day. The only thing in life that you can control is the way that you react to change. The people that shine the brightest light are those who never allow people or circumstances to dictate their attitude or the tone of their day. Find statements that empower you and then "never, never, never give up!"

- **Positive Self-Talk:**

  Self-talk can be either very detrimental to your mental and physical health. You need to make the choice to find ways to talk to yourself in a positive and healthy way. If you fail at a task, tell yourself that you're happy that you attempted the task. Reward yourself for trying instead of punishing yourself for failing. People will often hear me reciting the "Our Father" or "Hail Mary" when I am struggling. I try to replace any negative self-talk with prayers, or I discuss in my head ways that I can do something in a more positive manner the next time, which might increase my level of effectiveness and enjoyment of a task. This relates to everything in your life and not just your exercise or workout routine. Having a bad day at work, talk to yourself about the tasks that you accomplished and the positive conversations you've had with your co-workers today.

Lastly – NEVER engage in judgmental self-talk about others. What you might not notice is that your body and your mind act out what you think. You may be friendly and positive to someone you think less of, but your mind acts out those thoughts that can be consciously or subconsciously picked up by the person you are self-talking about. Be a positive person and a positive light on the world.

Visualize Your Goals:

Visualization is a powerful technique that can enhance motivation and goal attainment. Write out your goals in sentence form and the present or future tense that you have already met your goals. Read them each day while you warm up, cool down and just before bed. Let your subconscious do some of the work!

Example: I am working out 20 minutes a day including my warmup and cool downs. I enjoy sitting on the floor stretching each night while watching television. Each day I eat 6 – 8 smaller meals. I enjoy trying to get more fruits and vegetables into my diet. Each week we walk, playing tennis (or pickleball) and parking farther away from appointments and taking the stairs instead of the elevator.

Read this each day with a positive attitude and in a happy tone.

- **Creating Mental Images:**

  When our kids were younger, we pulled out a stack of old magazines and 3 foamcore boards. We asked the kids to cut out images and saying that show the type of person they are at the top of the board and at the bottom of the board hey type of person they want to become. When they were done, we asked them to explain the images and saying and why they were important to them. Saying what you think out loud helps to reaffirm those thoughts. Each of our kids kept those in their room and looked at them often. The conversations they would have when their friends would visit would not only reaffirm their commitment to who they wanted to be, but they also shared with their friends who supported them on their journeys. Create a positive mental image of who you wish to be and put them all over your life and look at them often.

- **Linking Effort to Outcomes:**

You know the old saying, "No Pain, No Gain." Well, with low impact exercise, there is pain, not like you would get if you were running a marathon, or a triathlon, or lifting heavy weights, but there is pain. When you go from nothing to a new program there is going to be pain. The pain is temporary, but the results will last a lifetime. There are so many benefits to living an active lifestyle. Such as clarity of thought, better breathing, less effort required to achieve daily tasks. Climbing stairs with a laundry basket will no longer feel like a chore. As you track your food intake, heart rate and blood pressure you will begin to see the outcomes of your effort.

Reward Your Progress:

I like to think of these rewards in immediate, near, and far term rewards. It takes 30 days of daily work for it to become a habit. Reward yourself each day the first week for eating right and working out. Then reward yourself at the end of the 2nd week for meeting that milestone. Then week #3, and the end of the first month. Have a calendar that shows what your goals are or each day. Cross them off and pat yourself on the back each day. Find an accountability partner who will hold you accountable to completing your tasks. Post your first 30-day goal on your Facebook page and then post your accomplishments each day for accountability and praise from your family and friends. Set up 3, 6, 9, and 12 month rewards that you are working towards. Remember that when you start on the journey, it is the path just as much as the goal. If you don't hit your goal, but you achieve significant results along the way, that is still something to celebrate. Just realign your goals based on what you learned and keep working.

Motivational Synergy:

Motivation is a dynamic force that can be sustained through a thoughtful blend of inspirational quotes, daily affirmations, encouragement from others and rewards. This synergy ensures that you are not only inspired but also equipped with practical tools to stay motivated on your fitness journey.

NOTES:

Chapter Eleven

Consultation with Professionals

Collaboration: Partnering with Healthcare Providers

The Importance of Collaboration

Your health journey is a collaborative effort, and this chapter underscores the significance of partnering with healthcare professionals. We'll delve into the benefits of engaging in open conversations with your primary care physician and specialists, forging a partnership that ensures a comprehensive approach to your well-being. Collaboration becomes a cornerstone in your quest for a healthier, more vibrant life.

Expert Insights: Invaluable Guidance

Discover the wealth of insights that collaboration with healthcare providers can bring. From personalized exercise recommendations to a deeper understanding of your unique health needs, expert guidance becomes an invaluable resource on your wellness journey. By weaving healthcare expertise into your exercise program, you empower yourself with the knowledge and support necessary for a safe and effective routine.

Regular Check-ins:

Emphasize the importance of ongoing communication with healthcare professionals. Regular check-ins provide an opportunity to discuss progress, address concerns, and make adjustments to the exercise program based on evolving health needs.

Seeking professional guidance ensures a holistic approach to health and minimizes potential risks associated with exercise, especially for individuals with specific health considerations.

NOTES:

Chapter Twelve

Resources

Reputable Sources of Aortic Aneurysm Information Websites:

https://www.heart.org/en/health-topics/aortic-aneurysm

https://www.webmd.com/search?query=aortic%2Baneurysm

https://johnritterfoundation.org/support-and-resources/

https://vascular.org/patients-and-referring-physicians/conditions/abdominal-aortic-aneurysm

https://pages.clevelandclinic.org/aortic-aneurysm-index-2.html?utm_source=google_ppc&utm_medium=cpc&utm_campaign=Heart+-+Aortic+Aneurysm+-+General+-+Region+1,+2,+3,+4,+5,+6,+7,+8,+9&utm=abdominal%20aortic%20aneurysm&gclid=CjwKCAiA98WrBhAYEiwA2WvhOmi8irbD16fZa_35TA9eH9Ap37QNgoK2lfPTd8Zri2fp0HI7lGfrzxoCzSQQAvD_BwE&gclsrc=aw.ds

https://www.mayoclinic.org/diseases-conditions/abdominal-aortic-aneurysm/diagnosis-treatment/drc-20350693

https://www.nhlbi.nih.gov/health/aortic-aneurysm/treatment

https://www.cdc.gov/heartdisease/aortic_aneurysm.htm

Mediterranean Diet Resource Websites:

https://www.mayoclinic.org/healthy-lifestyle/nutrition-and-healthy-eating/in-depth/mediterranean-diet/art-20047801

https://my.clevelandclinic.org/health/articles/16037-mediterranean-diet

https://www.heart.org/en/healthy-living/healthy-eating/eat-smart/nutrition-basics/mediterranean-diet

https://www.webmd.com/diet/a-z/the-mediterranean-diet

D.A.S.H. Diet Resource Websites:

https://www.mayoclinic.org/healthy-lifestyle/nutrition-and-healthy-eating/in-depth/dash-diet/art-20048456

https://www.webmd.com/hypertension-high-blood-pressure/dash-diet

https://www.heart.org/en/health-topics/high-blood-pressure/changes-you-can-make-to-manage-high-blood-pressure/managing-blood-pressure-with-a-heart-healthy-diet

https://www.kidney.org/atoz/content/Dash_Diet

https://www.eatright.org/health/health-conditions/cardiovascular-health-heart-disease-hypertension/dash-diet-reducing-hypertension-through-diet-and-lifestyle

Chapter Thirteen

Disclaimer

The information provided in this book is for general informational purposes only and is not intended to be a substitute for professional medical or fitness advice. The author and publisher are not healthcare professionals, and the content within this book should not be considered as professional advice.

Before beginning any exercise program or making significant changes to your lifestyle, it is recommended that you consult with a qualified healthcare professional. The exercises, dietary recommendations, and health strategies outlined in this book may not be suitable for everyone, and individual results may vary.

The author and publisher disclaim any liability, loss, or risk incurred as a consequence, directly or indirectly, of the use and application of any content within this book. Readers are advised to use their discretion and judgment, taking into consideration their personal health conditions and limitations.

Participation in physical activities carries inherent risks, and readers are urged to ensure they are in good health before engaging in any exercise program presented in this book. If at any point during the activities outlined in this book you feel unwell or experience discomfort, it is imperative to stop immediately and seek medical attention.

The author and publisher are not responsible for any injuries, accidents, or health complications that may arise from the use of the information in this book. By choosing to follow the advice and practices outlined herein, readers acknowledge that they do so at their own risk.

Before commencing this or any exercise program, it is advisable to consider acquiring an exercise watch or heart rate monitor that can be regularly consulted during your workout sessions. Prior to initiating any fitness regimen, it is strongly recommended to consult with your doctor or cardiologist for guidance and advice regarding appropriate heart rate ranges for low-impact exercises.

About the Author

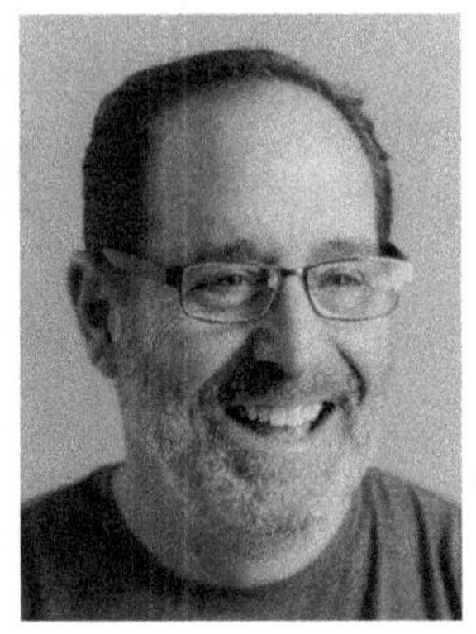

Embarking on a life of adventure and exploration, Scott Schmidt has spent most of his adult life traversing the globe, cultivating his expertise in promotional marketing sales alongside such clients such as Harley-Davidson and Snap-on Tools. His remarkable journey has taken him from the serene Buddhist Temples to the opulent French Monasteries, from the iconic Sydney Opera House to the exhilarating European Rally in Faaker See, Austria. Scott's travels extend to the heart-pounding F1 races in Shanghai and Singapore, as well as motorcycle rides weaving through the picturesque landscapes of Monaco, Italy, Switzerland, the United Kingdom, France, Germany, Canada, and across the United States, including the legendary Sturgis and Daytona events, and cruising into the Harley-Davidson Anniversaries in Milwaukee from both Las Vegas, NV, and Sarasota, FL. Whether on the saddle of a motorcycle or gazing out of an airplane window, Scott has truly witnessed the world in all its splendor.

Beyond his globetrotting adventures, Scott finds joy in a myriad of activities, including snow skiing, fishing (both open water and ice fishing), gardening, beer making, cooking, grilling, smoking foods, and even navigating the skies in small planes. A man of action, Scott's routine once included daily walks spanning 8 to 10 miles, bicycle rides, and rigorous workouts – until one pivotal morning at the age of 58.

Facing a sudden onset of atrial fibrillation (aFib), Scott spent 4.5 hours with his heart racing at marathon-like intensity. Exhausted and concerned, a visit to the emergency room revealed an unexpected discovery – an aortic aneurysm, a condition he shared with his maternal Grandmother. Although the aneurysm was initially small, the imperative became finding a way to maintain an active lifestyle without risking an increase in its size. This revelation marked the beginning of a new chapter for Scott.

In this book, Scott candidly shares his journey of self-discovery and resilience, navigating the challenges of living with an aortic aneurysm. Drawing from personal experiences, trial and error, as well as a wealth of knowledge gained from extensive reading, online resources, and videos since his diagnosis in 2022, Scott offers valuable insights, practical advice, and inspiration for others facing similar health challenges. *"Aneurysm-Friendly Exercise Guide"* serves as a testament to Scott's determination to live life to the fullest, embracing both the thrill of adventure and the resilience required to overcome unexpected obstacles.

Credits

Cover Photo:

Image by <a href="https://www.freepik.com/free-photo/full-shot-happy-friends-sitting-bench_18892714.htm#page=2&query=60%20year%20old%20coupl es%20playing%20with%20grandchildren&position=1&from_view=s earch&track=ais&uuid=5036b217-4004-4d99-a111-93b71e377461">Freepik</a>

Photo of Author:

Nathanial Schmidt Photography - www.nathanialschmidt.com

Images and Illustrations:

Abdominal Aortic Aneurysm – Chapter 3 – Society for Vascular Surgery - https://vascular.org/patients-and-referring-physicians/conditions/abdominal-aortic-aneurysm

Thoracic Aortic Aneurysm – Chapter 3 – Cleveland Clinic - https://my.clevelandclinic.org/health/diseases/17552-aorta-thoracic-aortic-aneurysm